Julieta Melendi

Outlines of stress-related mental disorders in health care workers

Julieta Melendi

Outlines of stress-related mental disorders in health care workers

during the COVID-19 pandemic in Argentina

ScienciaScripts

Imprint

Any brand names and product names mentioned in this book are subject to trademark, brand or patent protection and are trademarks or registered trademarks of their respective holders. The use of brand names, product names, common names, trade names, product descriptions etc. even without a particular marking in this work is in no way to be construed to mean that such names may be regarded as unrestricted in respect of trademark and brand protection legislation and could thus be used by anyone.

Cover image: www.ingimage.com

This book is a translation from the original published under ISBN 978-620-3-87815-8.

Publisher:
Sciencia Scripts
is a trademark of
Dodo Books Indian Ocean Ltd., member of the OmniScriptum S.R.L Publishing group
str. A.Russo 15, of. 61, Chisinau-2068, Republic of Moldova Europe
Printed at: see last page
ISBN: 978-620-4-12371-4

Outlines of stress-related mental disorders in health care workers during the COVID-19 pandemic in Argentina.

Julieta Melendi

Summary

This paper addresses the impact of the COVID-19 pandemic on stress-related mental disorders in hospital staff caring for patients with suspected or confirmed coronavirus in Argentina. To this end, research on mental disorders diagnosed in health workers who worked in hospitals that dealt with epidemic diseases such as SARS, MERS or Ebola is analyzed. In turn, the stress experienced by health workers when caring for suspected or confirmed COVID-19 patients is examined. Finally, it is proposed that Argentine regulations be brought into line with World Health Organization (WHO) and International Labour Organization (ILO) guidelines on the subject.

Keywords: stress - health workers - COVID-19

Descriptions of mental disorders associated with stress among health professionals during the Covid 19 pandemic in Argentina.

Summary

This paper addresses the impact of the COVID-19 pandemic on stress-related mental disorders in health professionals working in hospitals responsible for the care of patients with suspected or confirmed coronavirus in Argentina. To this end, research was conducted on mental disorders diagnosed in health professionals working in hospitals where other epidemic diseases such as SARS, MERS or Ebola were treated, and the stress experienced by health professionals caring for patients with suspected or confirmed COVID-19 was also studied. Finally, an Argentine regulation should be aligned with World Health Organization (OMS) and International Labour Organization (OIT) guidelines regarding this issue.

Palavras-chave: Stress- Pessoal de Saude- COVID-19

Sketches of stress-related mental disorders among health workers during the Covid 19 pandemic in Argentina.

Abstract

This paper addresses the impact of the COVID-19 pandemic on stress-related mental disorders in hospital staff responsible for the care of patients with suspected or confirmed coronavirus in Argentina. To this end, research will be conducted on mental disorders diagnosed in health workers who have performed their work in hospitals where epidemic diseases such as SARS, MERS or Ebola have been treated. At the same time, the stress of health workers caring for suspected or confirmed COVID-19 patients will be studied. Finally, it is proposed to harmonize Argentine regulations with World Health Organization (WHO) and International Labour Organization (ILO) guidelines.

Keywords: stress- health personnel- COVID-19

I. Introito

This paper addresses the impact of the COVID-19 pandemic on stress-related mental disorders in hospital staff caring for patients with suspected or confirmed coronavirus in Argentina.

In this sense, we adopt the World Health Organization (WHO, 2006) definition for the term "health worker", which defines it as "a person engaged in a paid activity whose direct or indirect aim is to promote or improve the health of the population" (cited in PAHO/WHO, 2013, p. 13).

Our research is relevant to the legal world because of the higher right at stake, namely the right to health of both the health professionals who perform their duties during the health crisis and the patients who may be victims of the symptoms of the stress-related mental disorders from which the former suffer or may suffer.

Therefore, we will focus on the analysis of the characteristics and symptoms of work-related stress, burnout syndrome and post-traumatic stress disorder. At the same time, we will look at previous research on mental disorders diagnosed in healthcare workers who have worked in hospitals with suspected or confirmed patients with epidemic diseases such as SARS, MERS, or Ebola, and we will examine recent research on the stress reported by healthcare workers caring for suspected or confirmed COVID-19 patients.

In turn, we will analyze the different factors listed by the International Labor Organization and the World Health Organization (ILO/WHO, 2020, pp. 70 and 71) as having sufficient potential to cause different stress-related mental disorders during health crises, making a comparative analysis with the current situation in Argentina.

Finally, we will address the Argentine legislation on stress and propose a reform of the list of occupational diseases established by the National Executive. To this end, the existing benefits and the corresponding consequences of our position will be examined.

II. The right to health

a. National and international protection

Health is a fundamental human right. But what are we talking about when we talk about human rights? As Antonio Truyol y Serra (1968) stated:

> To say that there are "human rights" or "rights of man" in our historical-spiritual context is tantamount to asserting that there are fundamental rights that man possesses by the very fact of being man, by his own nature and dignity: rights that are inherent in him and which, far from arising from a concession by political society, must be consecrated and guaranteed by it (quoted in Bidart Campos, 1989, p. 16).

In Argentina, its protection is guaranteed by articles 33, 41, 42 and 75(22) of the Argentine Constitution. In turn, the right to health is expressly enshrined in various human rights instruments enshrined in the Constitution, such as the following: The Universal Declaration of Human Rights of 1948 (article 25); the American Declaration of the Rights and Duties of Man of 1948 (article 11); the International Convention on the Elimination of All Forms of Racial Discrimination of 1965 (article 5, paragraph (e), subparagraph IV); the Convention on the Elimination of All Forms of Discrimination against Women of 1979 (article 11, paragraph 1, subparagraph (f)); the Convention on the Rights of the Child of 1989 (article 24); and the Convention on the Rights of Persons with Disabilities of 2006 (article 25).

It should be noted that the 1966 International Covenant on Economic, Social and Cultural Rights recognizes in Article 12 the right to physical and mental health as a human right and as a right of a worker. It states that "The States Parties to the present Covenant recognize the right of everyone to the enjoyment of the highest attainable standard of physical and mental health" and refers to the measures to be taken to ensure the effectiveness of this right:

> b. Improving all aspects of industrial hygiene and the environment; c. Prevention, treatment and control of epidemic, endemic, occupational and other diseases; d. Creation of conditions ensuring medical care and medical services for all in case of illness.

Accordingly, Article 14a of the national Constitution guarantees workers decent and just working conditions and stipulates that work is protected by law.

As regards the protection of workers' mental health, the International Labour Organization recognizes and protects this right through various Conventions, including Occupational Safety and Health Convention No. 155, 1981, and Recommendation No. 164, which promote the development of occupational safety and health policies to protect workers' physical and mental health; Occupational Health Services Convention No. 161, 1985, and Recommendation No. 171, which define the role of occupational health services in promoting workers' physical and mental health.

Of note is ILO Recommendation No. 194 on the List of Occupational Diseases, as updated in 2010, which for the first time includes mental and behavioural disorders, including post-traumatic stress disorder and other mental or behavioural disorders that are not covered when there is a scientifically proven direct link between exposure to risk factors at work and the worker's mental or behavioural disorders.

Article 17 of the 1998 Mercosur Social and Labour Declaration provides not only for the right of workers to a healthy environment, but also to the preservation of their physical and mental health, and obliges States to implement measures to prevent occupational accidents and diseases.

II.   b. Why is it necessary to protect the mental health of health workers?

During the COVID-19 pandemic, the importance of health workers in coping with the emergency became apparent. The International Labour Organization (ILO, 2009) emphasizes that "the protection of the worker against sickness, whether occupational or non-occupational ... is not only a labour right, but a fundamental human right and one of the ILO's main objectives, as set out in its Constitution" (p. 5).

A report conducted by the World Health Organization (WHO, 2006) prior to the pandemic, which examined the reality of the health workforce, concluded that approximately four million additional health workers would be needed in 57 Member States to meet the health needs of the population (cited in PAHO/WHO, 2013, p.64).

Given the inadequate human resources available prior to the disaster, it is a logical consequence that staff dealing with coronavirus patients are not adequately protected, leading to staff turnover. Stress leads to increased absenteeism, less time for staff to perform their duties, lower worker performance and development, more errors and accidents leading to litigation against the facility and staff (WHO, 2004, p. 9).

Similarly, in agreement with Antonio Lozano-Vargas (2020), we believe that neglecting the mental health of health workers affects patients' care, their "clinical understanding or decision-making ability, which could hinder the fight against COVID-19 infection" and "has a significant impact on their well-being and quality of life" (p. 51).

In this context, Jenny Firth-Cozens and Joanne Greenhalgh (1997) conducted a study in which they examined the opinions of 225 hospital doctors and general practitioners using anonymous questionnaires and analysed the relationship between work-related stress and the way they cared for their patients. It found that 82 of them had incidents where they felt that symptoms of stress had negatively affected the care they gave to their patients. When asked how the stress affected them, half of the respondents referred to decreased care, 40% expressed irritability or anger, seven percent reported serious errors that did not result in death, while two resulted in the death of the patient. Among the causes, 57% cited fatigue, 28% work overload, 8% depression or anxiety, and 5% the effects of alcohol (p. 1017).

Firth-Cozens (2020) asserts that stressed medical personnel have been shown to be more prone to error and less compassionate toward their patients (p. 2). He also notes difficulties with memory, decision-making, loss of concentration, and increased irritability that predispose to alcohol and other drug abuse (Firth-Cozens and Cornwell, 2019, p. 6).

However, when health professionals suffer from burnout syndrome, Rosa Gómez Esteban (2004) points out that they become "less sensitive, compassionate and even aggressive towards patients, with a distant, cynical treatment and a tendency to blame them for the problems they suffer" (p. 3104).

All of the factors that cause stress in health care workers during a pandemic, if left untreated, can lead to low self-esteem, distress, disinterest, and apathy (Gómez-Esteban, 2004, p. 3105).

Stress-related mental disorders cause anxiety and complicate relationships with patients, relatives and colleagues. When relationships between staff become conflictual, this not only affects the institution, but also the healing process of patients (Gómez-Esteban, 2004, 3108).

For Herbert Freudenberger (1974), burnout syndrome is even contagious, as those "who suffer from it can infect others with their fatigue, despair, and cynicism, so that the organization can fall into a general dejection in a short time" (as cited in Souto and Martín, 2008, p. 44).

Stress-related mental disorders, in turn, are suicidal to the extreme for medical personnel. In this sense, several authors, based on different studies, point to high suicide rates among physicians (Gómez-Esteban, 2004, p. 3104).

III. Stress-related mental disorders

The International Labour Office (1984) defines psychosocial factors as those which.

> Interactions between work, its environment, job satisfaction, and organizational conditions on the one hand, and the worker's skills, needs, culture, and personal situation outside of work on the other, all of which can influence health, job performance, and satisfaction through perception and experience (p. 12).

Psychosocial factors are descriptive, as they refer to the structure of the organization, i.e. culture, environment, interpersonal relationships, while psychosocial risk factors are predictive, i.e. they refer to the inherent potential of working conditions to affect workers' health. Thus, psychosocial risk factors can have an unfavorable impact on career development by causing stress-related mental disorders and, consequently, affecting workers' quality of life (Uribe-Prado et al., 2014, p. 1555).

The International Labour Organization (ILO, 2016) gives examples of the inclusion of stress-related disorders in the list of occupational diseases in each country. For example, it mentions that they could be grouped under post-traumatic stress disorder, mental disorders, burnout, diseases caused by psychosocial factors or work-related stress (p. 16).

Although the ILO proposes to include them under each of the names given, a brief distinction is made below between work-related stress, burnout and post-traumatic stress disorder, with the main features and symptoms of each name given not only for academic reasons but also so that they will be included in general terms under the name "stress-related mental disorders" when the list of occupational diseases is amended in the future. This is to ensure that the various syndromes that may occur are included rather than excluded.

a. Stress at work

García-Moran and Gil-Lacruz (2016) state that it is difficult to define stress, as many diseases have identical symptomatology as a syndrome (p. 15).

Souto and Martín (2008) define it as "the organism's nonspecific adaptive response to change, demands, pressures, challenges, or threats" and explain that when it occurs in the workplace, it is referred to as "work-related stress" (pp. 11 and 12).

Depending on the response given by each person, a distinction can be made between eustress and distress: The former is "a stimulation that the subject is able to deal effectively with basically positive consequences, and 'distress', which would be an excessive experience beyond the subject's control" (Ovalles and Uribe, 2012, p. 69).

Specifically for us, the World Health Organization (2004) defines work-related stress as "a person's response to work demands and pressures that are not commensurate with his or her knowledge and skills and that test his or her ability to cope with the situation" (p. 3).

In this sense, the National Institute of Occupational Safety and Health (NIOSH, 1999) highlights that the main stressor is work, because "sometimes there is a lack of positive experiences, and in other cases there is an excess of negative aspects of work, such as lack of safety, risky or dangerous situations, or an excessive number of working hours" (cited by García-Moran and Gil-Lacruz, 2016, p. 17).

Work-related stress has both physical and psychological negative effects on those affected. Among the physical symptoms, Universidad Católica Boliviana San Pablo (2007) highlights: "tachycardia, increased blood pressure, sweating, changes in breathing rhythm, increased muscle tension, increased blood sugar, increased basal metabolic rate, increased cholesterol, inhibition of the immune system" (p. 60). García-Moran and Gil-Lacruz (2016) add:

> Incidence of irritable bowel syndrome, nervous tics, obesity and overweight, hair loss and dandruff, irregular menstruation, heart disease, ... Bruxism, cold hands and feet, muscle tension, loss of appetite or increased appetite, diarrhea or constipation, insomnia, stuttering, skin disorders (acne, rosacea, urticaria, wrinkles, sagging, dyshidrosis, psoriasis, oral herpes), fatigue and dry mouth (p. 16).

Mercedes Bueno and Sergio Barrientos-Trigolos (2020) mention among the psychological symptoms various depressive symptoms, including:

> Hopelessness, despair, sadness, tearfulness, altered appetite, irritability, frustration, feelings of worthlessness, loss of pleasure in usual activities, difficulty thinking, concentrating, deciding, and remembering, fatigue, or lack of energy (p. 2).

Stress, in turn, "manifests itself in other psychological states: e.g., tension, anxiety" (Robbins and Judge, 2009, p. 642). It also highlights "feelings of worry, indecision, poor concentration, disorientation, moodiness, hypersensitivity to criticism, and feelings of lack of control"

(Universidad Católica Boliviana San Pablo, 2007, p. 60).

Stress is also claimed to cause various behavioural changes in individuals, such as "altered eating habits, increased smoking and alcohol consumption, rapid speech, restlessness and sleep disturbances" (E. M. de Croon et al, 2004, cited in Robbins and Judge, 2009, p. 642).

b. Burnout Syndrome

The burnout syndrome (translated from English as "being burnt out" or defined as "exhaustion") has been studied several times among healthcare workers. It was first defined in 1974 by Herbert Freudenberger in a study of health care workers in hospitals in the United States, and was further elaborated in 1986 by Cristina Maslach, who also studied the nursing professions (Paredes, Sanabria-Ferrand, 2008, cited in PAHO/WHO, 2013, p. 26).

Different authors agree that burnout is a consequence of chronic work-related stress (Martínez-Pérez, 2010, p. 44). In this sense, Maslach and Jackson (1981) conceptualize it as:

> a reaction to chronic work stress that leads to feeling emotionally exhausted, developing negative activities and feelings toward the people with whom one works (depersonalization activities), and processes of devaluing one's professional role (as cited in Carlín and Garcés de los Fallos Ruiz, 2010, p. 170).

Therefore, Cary Cherniss (1982) states that in burnout there is a transition in which the sufferer attempts to psychologically adapt to the stress in four phases. In the first phase, which he calls "stress," there is some instability between the demands of the job and the resources available to the worker to respond. In the second stage, called "exhaustion," the worker responds emotionally to this instability by exhibiting various symptoms such as restlessness, nervousness, anxiety, fatigue, or exhaustion. In the preliminary stage to burnout, he then locates the "coping phase", in which the employee's behaviour changes and a distant or indifferent treatment of patients sets in (quoted from Martínez-Pérez, 2010, p. 49).

For Schaufeli (1999), burnout is similar to stress and consists of three key areas: a decreased sense of personal efficacy, emotional exhaustion, and depersonalization (as cited in Firth-Cozens and Cornwell, 2009, p. 6). For Firth-Cozens and Cornwell (2009), depersonalization involves the development of negative perceptions about patients and is the area that is likely to limit compassion or produce cruelty in interactions with patients (p. 6).

According to Maslach and Jackson (1986), the symptomatology of burnout syndrome manifests itself in three areas:

> (a) burnout or emotional exhaustion, defined as fatigue and exhaustion that can manifest mentally and physically, with an emotional sense of not being able to give more of oneself to others; (b) cynicism or depersonalization, as the set of negative feelings, attitudes, and reactions that a person develops to remain distant and cold toward others, especially toward the recipients of one's work; and c) low self-actualization or performance dissatisfaction, characterized by a painful disillusionment with the meaning of one's life and with personal achievements; disappointment with work, feelings of failure, and low self-esteem are often its components (Gil-Monte, 2005; Maslach, Schaufeli, and Leiter, 2001; Uribe-Prado, 2008, cited by Uribe-Prado et al. 2014, S. 1555).

Finally, Buendía and Ramos (2001) divide burnout symptoms into four types: emotional, cognitive, behavioral, and social. Among the first, they include negativity, lack of hope and patience, disappointment, extinction of feelings, and again depression and helplessness, both of which appear in the above description of work-related stress. Cognitive symptoms include loss of skills, resourcefulness and attention, exacerbated criticism and altered self-perception. Behavioral symptoms include lack of organization, avoidance of responsibility and decision making, absenteeism from work, and increased use of substances such as alcohol and drugs. Finally, the social symptom is characterized by isolation, avoidance of work, and conflict with people in the family, circle of friends, or work environment (as cited in Martínez 2010, p. 61).

c. post-traumatic stress disorder

Since health workers were declared indispensable by Decree No. 297/201 of the National Executive on 19/03/2020, they have experienced traumatic situations such as exposure to the virus, witnessing the death of patients, staff or family members due to the virus, fear, stigmatization by society, lack of personal protection measures, factors that we will analyze in detail in the following section. However, it should be noted that these experiences, if not processed or channeled, can lead to post-traumatic stress disorder.

The latter can be defined in this sense as:

> a set of symptoms that a person develops after witnessing, participating in, or hearing about a stressful and extremely traumatic event characterized by death or threat to their physical integrity or that of others (American Psychiatric Association, 2003, as cited in Abaz et al, 2016, p. 42).

In the same vein, the Superintendencia de Riesgos del Trabajo (SRT, 2017) states that:

> A severe psychotraumatic experience, such as an event that endangers one's life or personal integrity, or when one witnesses death or injury, or when the integrity of others is compromised, may produce a state of psychotic clinical expression through a posttraumatic stress mechanism, i.e., psychopathological imagery with altered appraisal of reality may emerge, such as psychotic depression or psychotic paranoid states in response to the event (p. 75).

[1] Available at: https://www.boletinoficial.gob.ar/detalleAviso/primera/227042/20200320.

According to the National Institute of Mental Health (NIH, 2020), symptoms of this syndrome begin to manifest three months after the traumatic or stressful events and must last for at least one month. It divides the symptoms into four types, namely: "intrusive memory" symptoms, which consist of frequent dreams related to the traumatic experiences, feelings of sadness, constant reminders of the events, and physical stress symptoms; "avoidance symptoms," by which one avoids remembering the events or being in the places where they occurred; "hypervigilance and reactivity symptoms," which include inattention, insomnia, irritability, anger, recklessness, or tension; finally, "cognitive symptoms" include difficulty remembering important details of the event, guilt, negativity, and isolation (pp. 1 and 2). 1 y 2).

IV.   Sources of stress in health crises

The International Labour Organization and the World Health Organization (ILO and WHO, 2020) state that workers in health crises and emergencies are exposed to a variety of stressors, both during and after their work. (S. 70-71).

In this context, a comparative study between health care workers from nine hospitals in Toronto, Canada, who treated patients during the SARS outbreak and health care workers from four hospitals in Hamilton who did not is worth highlighting. The former reported significantly higher levels of burnout, psychological distress and post-traumatic stress compared to the latter (Maunder et al., 2006, p. 1924).

A cross-sectional study conducted in different regions of China, surveying 1257 healthcare workers in 34 hospitals with fever clinics or wards for patients with COVID-19 from January 29 to February 3, 2020, found a high prevalence of mental health symptoms among healthcare workers treating patients with COVID-19.

For example, 50.4% reported symptoms of depression, 44.6% reported anxiety, 34% reported insomnia, and 71.5% reported anxiety. In particular, nurses, women, Wuhan workers, and frontline workers directly involved in the diagnosis, treatment, or care of patients with suspected or confirmed COVID-19 reported the most severe symptoms across all measures. The study concludes that among Chinese healthcare workers exposed to COVID-19, women, nurses, people in Wuhan, and frontline healthcare workers are at high risk for developing adverse mental health outcomes and may need psychological support or intervention (Lai et al., 2020).

Next, we will examine different factors cited by the ILO and OM S (2020) as having sufficient potential to cause stress-related disorders in health care workers in medical emergencies, either during their deployment (from section a. to section g.) or afterwards (section h.). In addition, we will conduct a comparative analysis between these and different studies conducted in previous epidemics, as well as recent studies on stress and the COVID-19 pandemic in different countries and the current situation in Argentina.

a. fear for their health, the health of their family members or the health of their work colleagues

The first factor that exposes health workers to stress, according to ILO and WHO (2020), is fear for their own health, the health of family members, or the health of colleagues. In a study that surveyed health workers in hospitals in Hunan Province during the outbreak of coronavirus disease between January and March 2020, the most important stressors were concern for their own safety, concern for their own family, and concern for patient mortality. Medical personnel aged 31-40 years were most concerned about transmitting the virus to their family, possibly because most of them had young children and living parents. From the responses to the questionnaires, the most important factor that helped to alleviate the medical staff's stress was the reassurance that the family was well, not infected with COVID-19, and not believed to be at risk of infection (Cai et al., 2020, p. 14).

b. Stigmatisation by society

When cases of COVID-19 began to spread around the world, it caused panic not only among health workers in particular, but also in society in general. The news from different parts of the world and its mass dissemination had a detrimental effect. The way they were communicated, emphasizing deaths and the number of contagions over the number of cases, had negative consequences (Bueno Ferrá and Barrientos-Trigo, 2020, p. 2). When the objective was to promote prevention, the fear generated in the population led to discrimination against health workers by some individuals. Thus, we witnessed the actions of individuals who went so far as to pressure or threaten [2]health workers living in their buildings to move out . We agree with Erving Goffman (1963) that "in the midst of epidemics, the selfish survival instinct comes to the surface, leading to the rejection of the other and being seen as a likely source of contagion" (cited by Monterrosa-Castro et al., 2020, p. 208).

In a study analyzing the symptoms and perceptions of Colombian general practitioners working in March 2020, 39% reported feeling discriminated against because they are health professionals. Those who conducted this research confirm that during epidemics, two sociological effects occur in relation to health professionals: Stigmatization and discrimination (Monterrosa-Castro et al, 2020, p. 208).

In this context, it is worth highlighting a study that analysed the 2014-2016 Ebola virus

---

[2] Serious threat to a doctor in Barrio Norte: "Find another place to live, you decide or I decide" (23/04/2020). Infobae. Retrieved from: https://www.infobae.com/sociedad/2020/04/23/grave-amenaza-a-un-medico-en-barrio- norte-buscate-otro-lugar-para-vivir-decidis-vos-o-decido-yo/

disease outbreak in West Africa and concluded that health workers were particularly affected by fear-related stigma in the population and that fear-related behaviours and stigma are common during epidemics (O'Leary et al, 2018, pp. 1 and 3).

This is significant in that health workers who have experienced discrimination or stigma during a pandemic may suffer 60% emotional distress (Nickell et al., 2004, as cited in Monterrosa-Castro et al., 2020, p. 208).

c. The pressure of assigned tasks and the long working day

According to a study conducted by the Pan American Health Organization (PAHO/WHO, 2012) prior to the pandemic, approximately 20% of health workers in Argentina worked more than 48 hours per week (p. 36). On the other hand, the report highlights that 58% of nurses and 60% of physicians perceived the activities assigned to them as complex (p. 54) and the workload as high in terms of pace, intensity and shifts (p. 73). In addition, it is worth noting that 72% of Argentine physicians and 70% of Argentine nurses consider that they are regularly confronted with stressful or emotionally demanding tasks (p. 55).

Christiane Wiskow and Maren Hopfe[3] point out that there are several ways to protect health workers during the COVID 19 pandemic, including controlling assigned work hours. They point out that in crisis situations, health care workers must work under unusual conditions; they emphasize that in order to cope with the reality in which we find ourselves, many health care workers are engaged in caregiving, working long hours and getting little sleep. They say that this situation is exacerbated by their personal lives, in which they have to take care of their children because many educational institutions have been closed, or family members who are being cared for by them. Finally, they stress the need to provide them with rest periods so that workers can balance their work and personal lives.

Along these lines, a study assessing the psychological impact and coping strategies of frontline medical personnel in Hunan finds that frontline medical personnel in China have experienced an increase in workload, work hours, and increased psychological distress since the outbreak of coronavirus disease (COVID-19) in Hubei Province in November 2019 (Cai

---

[3] Wiskow C. and Hopfe M. (April 1, 2020), Five ways to protect health workers during the COVID-19 crisis. International Labour Organization. Available at: https://www.ilo.org/global/about-the- ilo/newsroom/news/WCMS_740405/lang--en/index.htm.

et al., 2020, p. 2).

In addition, the Pan American Health Organization (PAHO/WHO, 2020) calls on hospital leaders to initiate, promote, and accredit adherence to work breaks for health workers and to implement flexible work schedules for those caring for patients with suspected or confirmed COVID-19 and for those who have infected family members. It also emphasizes the need for health workers to spend time supporting each other as colleagues (p. 4).

d. push back self-care

Another factor considered sufficiently stressful by the ILO and WHO (2020) is the neglect of self-care, whether through lack of exercise, insufficient sleep or poor nutrition. However, we believe that the aforementioned behaviours are often a consequence of high workloads in the workplace.

A comparative study of health care workers who intervened and did not intervene during the SARS outbreak at Toronto and Hamilton hospitals in Ontario, Canada, which examined the long-term psychological and occupational effects, concluded that programs aimed at healthy lifestyles, diet, exercise, and smoking cessation can be important in supporting staff even after an outbreak (Maunder et al., 2006, p. 1931). Consequently, these habits are also a means of preventing PTSD.

e. Lack of basic safety equipment for personal protection

According to the ILO and WHO, another source of work-related stress for health workers during pandemic response is the lack of basic safety equipment for personal protection.

In the autonomous city of Buenos Aires, many hospitals lacked personal protective equipment to protect health workers from contracting COVID-19. For their part, professional risk insurers have failed to provide the necessary funds for this purpose.

Health workers were therefore forced to resort to the courts to obtain them. In short, we agree with Matías Molinaro (2019) that "the system, not as it is written in the law, but as it is actually practiced, exhibits the worker as the sole subject for demanding compliance ... due to the simple fact that he is the main victim of circumstances that endanger his health" (p. 309).

IV. e. 1. the case of the triage staff in the autonomous city of Buenos Aires

On 29/03/2020, the Ministry of Health of the Government of the City of Buenos Aires issued the "Protocol for the Treatment of Suspected and Confirmed Cases of Coronavirus (COVID-19)", which is constantly revised. [4]which is constantly revised.

The goal of the protocol is to rapidly identify suspected coronavirus cases in order to provide appropriate care to patients while taking all possible measures to investigate, prevent and control the virus.

The protocol requires that triage be performed each time a patient is admitted to the hospital. Thus, healthcare workers performing such tasks must identify patients who fall under the concept of a "suspected case" (as defined in the protocol itself), isolate those who are symptomatic, and take the necessary personal protective measures.

As Natalia Quezada Abascal (2020) notes, the protocol is criticized for requiring the provision of personal protective equipment to workers performing triage tasks only when there is a suspected case with certainty. In this way, health workers responsible for identifying and classifying cases entering the hospital do not have the necessary protective measures to safeguard their health (p. 1).

Notwithstanding the provisions of the Protocol, it must not be overlooked that there are hierarchically superior international and national regulations that impose the obligation to ensure health and safety in the workplace. However, we agree that the most reprehensible behaviour is that of employers who refuse to provide said health workers with personal protective equipment.

Analysis of the jurisprudence on the lack of provision of personal protective equipment to health workers during COVID-19 in the Autonomous City of Buenos Aires.

On 01/04/2020, the judge of the National Labor Court of First Instance No. 45, Rosalía Romero, granted an urgent precautionary measure requested by Carolina A. Cáceres, a nurse who works at the Hospital General de Acute Dr. Enrique Tornú. Cáceres, a nurse at Hospital General de Agudos Dr. Enrique Tornú, to establish safety elements to prevent the

---

[4] Available on the official website of the Government of the City of Buenos Aires at: https://www.buenosaires.gob.ar/sites/gcaba/files/pcero 5.pdf.

spread of the coronavirus and mitigate its effects [5]. This petition was filed against the Government of the City of Buenos Aires, which is obliged to provide the personal protective equipment in this case, and against the Provincia A.R.T. S.A., which has the duty to control it.

The Magistrate reiterates that the State has delegated the control and supervision of employers' health and safety standards to occupational risk insurers.

It mentions that one of the main objectives of the Occupational Risks Act (Act 24.557) is to reduce occupational accidents through risk prevention. It also highlights the role of risk insurers in the field of safety, as they must constantly carry out prevention and monitoring activities.

He points out that the right to life and health is enshrined in various international treaties, including the Universal Declaration of Human Rights, the American Convention on Human Rights, the American Declaration of the Rights and Duties of Man, the International Covenant on Civil and Political Rights and the International Covenant on Economic, Social and Cultural Rights, which in turn have constitutional status under Article 75, paragraph 22 of the National Constitution. At the same time, he points out that in this case the right to health and integrity of the human person has a double constitutional guarantee, since he is also a worker, relying on articles 14bis and 19 of the national Constitution.

The employer's duty to provide all elements and preventive measures to avoid the contagion of the disease by exposed workers, as well as the duty of prevention and control by the risk insurer, is based on the following legal framework: Article 75 of the L.C.T., Law 19.587, ILO Conventions No. 155 (on the safety and health of workers and its 2002 Protocol) and No. 187 (referring to the ILO Framework of Promotion of Safety and Health at Work), adopted by Laws 26.693 and 26.694, respectively, and the prevention obligation provided for in Article 1710 of the National Civil and Commercial Code.

Finally, the judge not only ordered the Government of the City of Buenos Aires to provide the

---

[5] "Cáceres, Carolina Alejandra v. Gobierno de la Ciudad de Buenos Aires s/ medida cautelar", JNTrab. N° 45, 01/04/2020. Available on the official website of the Dirección Nacional del Sistema Argentino de Información Jurídica, at. http://www.saij.gob.ar/juzgado-nacional-primera-instancia-trabajo-nacional-ciudad-autonoma-buenos-aires-caceres-carolina-alejandra-gobierno-ciudad-buenos-aires-amparo-fa20040004-2020-04-01/123456789-400-0400- 2ots-eupmocsollaf?

personal protective equipment and Provincia ART S.A. to provide the preventive and control means necessary for that purpose, each within 24 hours of service of the order, but also imposed fines of ten thousand pesos for each day of non-compliance with the order.

This solution appears to be the most appropriate, since, as the Magistrate argues, damage might otherwise be caused which would make subsequent reparation difficult or impossible.

The case law is consistent in this respect. In the case "Moya, Mónica Graciela y otros c/ GCBA y otros s/ medida cautelar autónoma" (Moya, Mónica Graciela y otros c/ GCBA y otros s/ medida cautelar autónoma), Expte. No. 3040/2020-0, of 17/04/20206, the Court of First Instance in Administrative and Fiscal Disputes No. 14, Secretariat No. 27, ordered the Municipality to provide the health personnel of Ramos Mejía Hospital with the unavoidable and adequate protective elements to prevent infection with the coronavirus, and Provincia ART S.A. is obliged to comply with the employer's hygiene, safety, control and surveillance regulations in accordance with the provisions of Law 24.557, to comply with the employer's hygiene, safety, control and surveillance regulations in accordance with the provisions of Law 24.557. This ruling was affirmed by Board I of the Board of Administrative, Fiscal and Consumer Appeals on 12/06/2020.

Moreover, on 14/05/2020, in the case "Correa, Rebeca Noemí c/ GCBA s/ Amparo-Public Employment-Others", Expte. N° 303030/2020-0, Chamber II of the Administrative, Fiscal and Consumer Appeals Chamber upheld[67] the precautionary measure issued by the judge of first instance ordering the Municipality to take the necessary measures to prevent the infection of employee Rebeca Noemí Correa, who works as a nurse in a public hospital, with COVID-19, and to immediately provide her with the adequate protection corresponding to the activity performed by the petitioner.

Finally, we agree with Alberto D. Chartzman Birenbaum (2020) that.

---

[6]"Moya, Mónica Graciela y otros c/GCBA y otros s/ medida cautelar autónoma", JNCAyT N° 14, 17/04/2020, Expte. N° 3040/2020-0, available on the official website of the Centro de Información Jurídica del Ministerio Público de la Ciudad de Buenos Aires, at: https://cijur.mpba.gov.ar/files/articles/1746/M.M-y-otros-contra-GCBA.pdf.

[7] "Correa, Rebeca Noemi c/GCBA s/Amparo- Empleo Público-Otros", CNCATyRC, Sala II, 14/05/2020, Expte. N° 3030/2020-0, available on the official website of the Department of Library and Jurisdiction of the Judicial Council of the City of Buenos Aires, at: http://juristeca.jusbaires.gov.ar/ics-wpd/exec/icswppro.dll?QB0=AND&QF0=IDFallo&QI0=41939&TN=Sumarios&DF=VerSumarios&RF=VerSumarios&DL=0&RL=0&MR=0&NP=4&AC=QBE QUERY&MF=msgSumarios.ini

The care of our health and that of others is not negotiable in the face of legal loopholes or mere mercantilist pretensions of voices that want to evade responsibility without thinking of the sensitivity and security that this inalienable value, which is part of human dignity, deserves (p. 10).

f. The desire to care for patients despite salary disputes

In this sense, there is a theory called "effort-reward" that analyzes the relationship between work and stress. It is based on the assumption that the environmental factor plays an important role at work. This factor includes organizational culture, the structure of the institution, the role assigned to job security, and compensation. On this basis, it concludes that when there is an imbalance between excessive work demands, whether quantitative (excessive working hours) or qualitative (intensity of assigned tasks), and the incentives provided to cope with them (remuneration), stress is generated in the employee (Palacios et al., 2014, p. 63).

For example, in the autonomous city of Buenos Aires, workers at ATE Capital Federal demonstrated in December for decent wages, disagreeing with the 23% annual wage parity proposed by the head of government. At the same time, workers at the Asociación de Licenciados en Enfermería (ALE) demanded "career recognition and salary increases". [8]

g. The enormous physical strain that personal protective equipment entails

Another factor cited by the ILO and WHO (2020) as sufficiently stressful for health workers in health crises is the high physical strain of wearing personal protective equipment. This can lead to exhaustion or dehydration.

In this regard, during the COVID-19 pandemic, health care workers must protect themselves with the following personal protective equipment: surgical mask, gown, gloves, eye protection and, if an aerosol-generating procedure is performed, the No. 95 mask recommended by the Argentine Ministry of Health[9]

---

[8] Health workers demonstrate for 'decent wages' and professional recognition (03/12/2020). Télam. Retrieved from: https://www.telam.com.ar/notas/202012/537315-paro-medicos-enfermeros-reclamo-salarios- dignos.html

[9]　　More information at: https://www.argentina.gob.ar/salud/coronavirus-COVID-19/recomendaciones-uso-epp#:~:text=Hygiene%20of%20Hands%2C%20Barbijo%20quir%20quir%3%BArgico,camisol%C3%ADn%2C%20guante s%2C%20protecci%C3%B3n%20ocular.

It is worth noting that in a study conducted by the Pan American Health Organization (PAHO/WHO, 2012) prior to the pandemic, 62% of nurses and 57% of medical personnel in Argentina reported that they regularly performed physically demanding tasks (p. 55).

h. Causes of stress after posting

For their part, the ILO and WHO (2020) cite bad memories of the experience, fear, and obstacles to reintegration into normal life as post-deployment factors (p. 71).

In a study conducted during the acute outbreak of SARS in Hong Kong, healthcare workers in high-risk situations not only reported psychological symptoms during the emergency, but 89% experienced secondary symptoms. For example, 71% reported fatigue, 59% reported health concerns, and 46% reported fear of social contact (Chua et al., 2004, p. 392).

On the other hand, another study conducted among 1 800 employees of Kyung Hee University Hospital in Gangdong who treated Middle East Respiratory Syndrome (MERS) patients during the May-December 2015 outbreak in Korea concluded that medical personnel who performed tasks related to the MERS virus had an increased risk of post-traumatic stress symptoms even after the time had passed (Lee et al., 2018, p. 123).

V. Current state of affairs in Argentina

a. Occupational Risks Act

Law 24.557 does not contain a concept of occupational disease, but is limited to stating that occupational diseases are those included in the list drawn up by the Executive in accordance with the procedure provided for in Article 40(3°) of the said law. This list specifies the risk agent, the pathologies, the exposure and the activities that may lead to the development of the occupational disease. None of the mental disorders related to stress are included in the above list.

Consequently, this illness and its consequences are in principle not compensable, with two exceptions provided for in Article 6(2)(b) and (c) of the Occupational Risks Act, namely whenever the Central Medical Commission establishes in a given case that the mental disorder was caused by a direct and proximate cause in the performance of work, excluding the influence of factors attributable to the worker or unrelated to work. Therefore, paragraph 3 of the said Article excludes occupational diseases caused by the worker's intent or by force majeure unrelated to the work, as well as incapacities of the worker prior to the employment relationship detected during the work examination.

It follows that Article 6(2)(b) and (c) provides for an administrative procedure limited to individual cases which does not entail any amendment of the list of occupational diseases in force, so that that list remains closed. Thus, each worker or his beneficiary must initiate the procedure by submitting a reasoned request to the Medical Tribunal Commission aimed at confirming the coincidence of risk agents, exposure, pathologies and activities with a direct causal effect in relation to the disease. Subsequently, the Medical Tribunal Commission will substantiate the application with a hearing of the person concerned, the employer and the occupational risk insurer and will issue a decision.

Notwithstanding the foregoing, any damage caused to the employee that is not recognized through the administrative channel provided for in the Occupational Risks Law leaves open the judicial channel for the recognition of the claim to which he is entitled by applying the rules of common law, so that in this case it is necessary to prove that the requirements of civil liability have been met. Thus, in the decision "Silva, Facundo Jesús c/ Unilever de

Argentina SA s/ Recurso de hecho" of 18.12.2007 [10], the Supreme Court of Argentina held that when an illness is not included in the closed list of Law 24.559, but the existence of a causal link with the work activity is recognized, the extra-systemic compensation under civil law is applicable. This is because the failure to compensate for illnesses that are not included in the list would violate the prohibition against harming another person enshrined in Article 19 of the National Constitution.

Specifically, in the decision "Papp Lourdes Mónica Andrea v Provincia ART S.A. s/ enfermedad accidente" (Papp Lourdes Mónica Andrea v Provincia ART S.A. s/ enfermedad accidente), the Fourth Chamber of the Mendoza Labour Court upheld the plaintiff's claim in a case of work-related stress suffered by a nurse who worked at "El Sauce" Hospital. [11]The plaintiff's claim was upheld because it was proven that she suffered from a psychiatric illness directly related to nursing work at the workplace, where she had to deal with former inmates of the male judicial ward B who constantly attacked her physical integrity by insulting her, abusing her, hitting her, setting her on fire and fleeing, among other things. Due to the repeated absence of police officers, she had to face this reality alone, resulting in sleeplessness, exhaustion and listlessness.

Due to this circumstance, she requested a change in her working hours in order to become calmer, but this was only granted for one month. Subsequently, she began to go to the psychiatric ward for various periods of time, because each time she returned to work, her situation remained unchanged. The situation was of such magnitude that the plaintiff continues to undergo psychiatric treatment and take medication. She was also diagnosed with depression, which manifests itself in anxiety, trepidation, irritability, pathological stress and insomnia. Therefore, her physician certified Claimant as having an abnormal life response with Grade IV depressive symptoms and a psychiatric disability of 30%, attributing

---

[10] "Silva, Facundo Jesús v. Unilever de Argentina SA s/ Recurso de hecho". CSJN, 18/12/2007, available on the official website of the National Directorate of the Argentine Legal Information System at: http://www.saij.gob.ar/corte-suprema-justicia-nacion-federal-ciudad-autonoma-buenos-aires-silva-facundo-jesus- unilever-argentina-sa-fa07000214-2007-12-18/123456789-412-0007-0ots-eupmocsollaf#.

[11] "Papp Lourdes Mónica Andrea c/ Provincia ART S.A. s/ enfermedad accidente". Chamber of Labour of Mendoza. Sala IV Unipersonal, 09/08/2019, available at: https://aldiaargentina.microjuris.com/2019/10/31/cuidar-de-los- demas-y-descuidarse-a-si-si-me-incapacidad-psiquica-que-padece-una-enfermera-a-raiz-de-las-situaciones-de-des- estres-vividas-en-el-hospital-en-el-que-bajaba/.

this condition to work-related stress.

The facts of the case show that the claimant filed the relevant complaint under Article 22 of Law 24.557 by letter, which was rejected. She also appealed to the Superintendence of Labour Risks at Medical Commission No. 4, which rejected the illness as non-culpable, although it found that the claimant suffered from abnormal constitutional personality, grade II.

When Provincia A.R.T. S.A. appeared on the record, it argued that the illness was uncaused and therefore outside any rate system.

The judge relied on the fact that although work-related stress is not included in the list of occupational diseases, the employer is responsible not only for compensation but also for prevention, as he is responsible for safety under Article 75 of the L.C.T.. This defines an occupational disease as "a disease which, although not specifically occupational, may be caused, aggravated or induced by conditions of hygiene and safety at work".

It relies on the precedent set by the "Borecki" case of the Second Chamber of the Mendoza Labour Court, which was upheld by the Mendoza High Court (file no. 72.153), in which it was confirmed that the promotion of a closed compensation system that excludes diseases not included in the list and causally linked to work violates the principle of non-compensation of others enshrined in Article 19 of the Magna Carta and the international instruments that have constitutional status (under Article 75, Section 22 of the National Constitution), such as the American Declaration of the Rights and Duties of Man and the American Convention on Human Rights. The precedent emphasized that the application of Law 24.557 in these cases would result in the person who should be held liable being exempted from liability, while the worker would have to bear the damage caused by his condition himself, in violation of the principle of equality enshrined in Article 16 of the National Constitution.

In view of the foregoing, the judge ordered Provincia A.R.T. S.A. to pay compensation in the amount of $315,939.87 for partial, permanent and definitive disability, noting that the fact that the plaintiff had received a risk surcharge pursuant to Resolution No. 2216 did not offset the compensation assessed on account of the mental disability suffered. Lastly, it declared Article 6, section 2 of Law 24,557 unconstitutional.

b. Prevention and organisational culture

Although the ILO and WHO (2020) make recommendations for reducing health workers' stress at work during health crises through individual, group, and organizational cultural practices (pp. 72-74), we agree with Gómez-Esteban (2004) that in addressing the issue of stress-related mental disorders, the focus is on the personal characteristics of the sufferer rather than the personal characteristics of the person suffering from stress. 72-74), we agree with Gómez-Esteban (2004) that in treating the issue of stress-related mental disorders, the focus is on the personal characteristics of the sufferer rather than the working conditions; although the former have an influence, we concur with the position of those who believe that working conditions are paramount in these assumptions (p. 3105). The institutional dynamics of the hospital are characterized by "dictatorial leadership, a constant increase in the pressure of care and responsibility, combined with a lack of autonomy and freedom of decision on the part of the physician" (Gómez-Esteban, 2004, p. 3102).

Given the prevailing situation in health care, we therefore disagree with the emphasis on the individual conditions of health care workers and the consequent insistence that it should be those who adopt stress prevention strategies. Answers given from an individualistic perspective may be helpful to those who show symptoms of stress, but are not meant to last as institutional involvement. Furthermore, this message is dangerous to say the least, as it would lead the professional to view the syndrome suffered as a purely individual matter, a personal failure, as he or she was unable to face the challenges of reality (Montgomery et al., 2019).

In addition, one study showed that working in overcrowded wards (bed occupancy of 10% or more above the recommended limit for six months) was related to the use of antidepressants by doctors and nurses; and the higher the ward bed occupancy, the more likely the use of antidepressants (Virtanen et al., 2008, cited by Firth-Cozens and Cornwell, 2009, pp. 7-8). This is significant considering that during the pandemic, several hospitals around the world collapsed to capacity.

On the other hand, although one of the objectives stated in article 1° paragraph 2° of Law 24.557 is the reduction of occupational accidents through prevention, since mental disorders related to stress are not included in the list of occupational diseases, it seems that the employer is not obliged to prevent them and the insurer of the occupational risk does not have the duty to control them. However, we agree with Julio A. Grisolía and Ernesto J. Ahuad (2019) that occupational stress should be treated as any risk to occupational health and safety, with the consequent obligation to conduct a periodic risk assessment. They define the latter as follows:

> the process by which the safety and health risks to workers exposed to hazards at work are assessed. It is a systematic examination of all aspects of the work, looking at what can cause injury or harm, whether these hazards can be eliminated and, if not, what preventive or protective measures should be introduced to control the risks.
>
> It is the basis for successful management of work-related stress and does not use different basic principles and processes from those used for other occupational risks (i.e. identifying risks and people at risk, assessing risks and ranking their importance, deciding on preventive measures, taking action, monitoring and reviewing) (pp. 282 and 283) (pp. 282 and 283).

In this sense, the International Labour Organization (ILO, 2020) states that in the situation we are in during the COVID-19 pandemic, essential workers are likely to be exposed to higher levels of stress and that therefore "related psychosocial factors in the workplace ... should be taken into account when examining the working conditions and safety of workers", suggesting that measures should be taken for the most vulnerable workers, among which it exclusively mentions health workers (p. 26).

VI. Relevant consequences of our position

Teresa Paz Koler and Norma Martín (2008) point out the difficulty of classifying stress as an occupational disease, since the factors at work in each worker are multicausal, regardless of the job they perform. Therefore, they cite as an important point in assessing whether stress constitutes an occupational disease the fact that the reality described by the worker is found in a large percentage of workers who have held the same job or performed the same tasks. It is important to consider "whether stress is the result of constant, difficult or impossible to avoid threats to the integrity, safety of one's own life or the lives of others caused by work performance" (cited in Álvarez-Chávez, 2008, pp. 59-60).

Following this analysis, and taking into account the situation before the pandemic, it is worth noting that in a comparative study conducted by the Pan American Health Organization (PAHO/WHO, 2012) on the working conditions and health of health personnel in Argentina, Brazil, Costa Rica and Peru, it was found that doctors and nurses in Argentina suffer from burnout in 59% and 55%, respectively, among the countries with the highest percentages (p. 73).

In another study by the Pan American Health Organization (PAHO/WHO, 2013), which surveyed health care workers in general facilities in the province of Buenos Aires Aires, 54.9% of workers reported suffering from stress, and of this percentage, the majority indicated that it was related to work in all or some cases. In addition, half of the workers reported a constant feeling of fatigue and more than a third reported sleep problems, irritability, physical fatigue, headaches and memory problems (p. 96).

We thus assume a complex situation from which it appears that health personnel in Argentina before the pandemic had at least the symptomatology of work-related stress. It should be noted, however, that these syndromes have been extensively studied in medical personnel. To such an extent that Firth-Cozens (2020) states that these problems will never disappear because health care is a responsible, inherently stressful profession and therefore systems are needed that recognize this fact and constantly work to solve these problems, for the benefit of doctors and their patients (p. 2).

This reality is exacerbated during health crises in general and during the COVID-19 pandemic in particular, so that in an article drawing parallels between the 2003 coronavirus outbreak and SARS, in terms of infectious cause, epidemiological characteristics, pattern of rapid transmission and inadequate preparedness of health authorities to deal with outbreaks, and considering the psychosocial impact of viral epidemics in general, highlights the need for urgent and timely treatment of outbreaks, The pattern of rapid transmission and the inadequate preparedness of health authorities to deal with outbreaks, as well as considering the psychosocial impact of viral epidemics in general, highlight the need for urgent and timely attention to the mental health of health workers through the development and implementation of mental health assessment, support, treatment and inclusion services (Xiang et al., 2020, S. 1). 228 y 229).

In this finding, taking into account that in different studies cited in this document, health professionals showed symptoms of stress during the COVID-19 pandemic and that, in turn, the risk factors that have sufficient potential to cause the aforementioned mental disorders increased, we consider that the stress-related illnesses of health professionals who worked in hospitals where patients with suspected or confirmed COVID-19 were treated from 19.03.2020 (date on which the disease was declared essential personnel in Argentina) were treated, should be included in the list of occupational diseases established by the National Executive in accordance with the procedure established in Article 40(3) of Law 24.557.

To this end, we consider it useful to group them under the general term "stress-related mental disorders", since, as we have studied, different syndromes appear depending on the intensity and duration of the stress or whether it manifests during or after the traumatic experiences. In this sense, we consider that the risk agent is the work itself, carried out during the pandemic.

Inclusion on the list is intended to enable health workers who have suffered a traumatic experience during the pandemic to obtain compensation for this occupational disease and its consequences. This would also avoid the need for each individual worker to go through the procedure provided for in Law 24.557 to have the illness recognised as an occupational disease before the Central Medical Commission.

In turn, this would reduce litigation as healthcare workers would no longer have to go to court to seek redress. In this sense, the need to litigate in order to obtain the right to which they are entitled is not only a factor that causes more stress, but can also worsen the mental health of the workers concerned, as it takes so long for them to enforce their right in court.

On the other hand, it should be noted that ILO Recommendation No. 194 on the list of occupational diseases that States should include in their lists included mental and behavioural disorders in the 2010 update [12]; that, in turn, WHO, through revision No. 11 of the International Classification of Diseases, included [13]burnout syndrome as an occupational phenomenon in the chapter entitled "Factors affecting the worker's state of health or health status".

Contact with health services, including reasons for which people contact health teams but which are not classified as diseases or medical conditions", which will come into force on 01.01.2022; and that the ILO (2020) has specifically recommended that both coronavirus and "post-traumatic stress disorder caused by exposure at work ... be considered as occupational diseases" (cited in Romualdi, 2020, p. 40), we consider that our proposed reform is the most appropriate way to bring the current regulations in line with the international guidelines.

Finally, we believe that maintaining the mental health of health workers will lead to an improvement in the quality of health services provided to society.

---

[12] Available in:
https://www.ilo.org/wcmsp5/groups/public/@.ed protect/@protrav/@.safework/documents/publication/wcms 12516 4.pdf.
[13] Available at: https://icd.who.int/browse11/l-m/en.

VII. CONCLUSIONS

The pandemic has accelerated many changes, but it has also brought other problems to the fore. It is worth highlighting the work of health workers who, despite the existing constraints, helped patients with suspected or confirmed COVID-19, overcoming various obstacles that put their health and lives at risk, as well as those of their relatives. Thus, we analyzed how, despite the lack of personal protective equipment, despite the discrimination and/or stigmatization they experienced, despite the various wage disputes, despite the long working hours, despite the physical and emotional burden of the health crisis we are going through, they continue to work to take care of the health and lives of the people who visit the hospital facilities. But who is looking after their health and lives? The national and international legal framework that recognizes health as a fundamental human right and guarantees the protection of workers' mental health is becoming moot in the face of these traumatic experiences.

Much has been written about the various stress-related mental disorders of healthcare workers. However, the C OVID-19 pandemic has exacerbated the situation. For example, in several studies reviewed, health care workers reported symptoms of stress-related mental disorders in both previous epidemics and the current pandemic.

Considering that stress-related mental disorders are not included as an occupational disease in the list established by the National Executive in accordance with the procedure established in article 40, paragraph 3, of Law 24.557, we consider that they should be included in relation to the work of health personnel who have worked in hospitals where patients with suspected or confirmed COVID-19 have been treated as of 03/19/2020 (the date on which it was declared essential personnel in Argentina).

The International Labour Organization (ILO, 2016) proposes examples for each state to include such mental disorders in the list of occupational diseases. Although it mentions that they could be included under the name of post-traumatic stress disorder, burnout, diseases caused by psychosocial factors or work-related stress, among others, we believe that they should be included in the list of occupational diseases under the general name of "stress-related mental disorders". In this sense, we consider that the risk agent is the work performed during the pandemic.

Among the benefits considered is that it would avoid the need for each individual health worker to go through the process of having these diseases recognised as occupational diseases before the Central Medical Commission, which is governed by Act 24.557. At the same time, this would reduce litigation by eliminating the need for health care workers to go to the courts to seek redress. In this sense, litigation over the right to which they are entitled not only leads to more stress, but may also worsen the mental health of the workers concerned in the time it takes to enforce rights through the courts.

Another advantage is the possibility of obliging employers and insurers of occupational risks to take various preventive measures (beyond risk assessment), and not only individual or group prevention strategies for employees. Maintaining the mental health of health workers will lead to improvements in the quality of health services provided to society. It has been shown that health professionals suffering from these syndromes become distant, insensitive, intolerant and even abusive towards their patients (Gómez-Esteban, 2004, p. 3104). As mentioned earlier, stress-related mental disorders increase absenteeism, affect worker performance and development, lead to a greater number of errors and accidents that can cause patient deaths, and consequently promote lawsuits against the institution and staff (WHO, 2004, p. 9).

Finally, it should be noted that ILO Recommendation No. 194 (2010 update) on the list of occupational diseases that States should include in their schedules included mental and behavioural disorders for the first time. Similarly, the WHO has included burnout syndrome as an occupational phenomenon in Revision No. 11 of the International Classification of Diseases, and the ILO (2020) has specifically recommended that post-traumatic stress disorder caused by pandemic work could be included in the list of occupational diseases (cited in Romualdi, 2020, p. 40). Therefore, there is no doubt that the reform we are formulating is guided by the tendency to seek harmonization with this normative framework.

BIBLIOGRAPHIC REFERENCES

- Abaz B., Babbino V., Volpi M., Orlando G. and Valdez P. (2016), "Estudio del estrés postraumático en personal de salud que ha participado en eventos con víctimas múltiples", *Revista argentina de medicina,* 4(9), 40-49, available at: http://revistasam.com.ar/index.php/RAM/article/view/67

- Álvarez-Chávez, V. H. (2008), *Ley de riesgos del trabajo: ley N° 24.557 y modificaciones. Comentada y anotada con jurisprudencia,* Editorial García Alonso.

- Bidart-Campos, G. J. (1989), *Teoría general de los derechos humanos,* Universidad Nacional Autónoma de México, Instituto de Investigaciones jurídicas, Ciudad Universitaria.

- Bueno-Ferrán M., Barrientos-Trigo S. (2020), "Caring for the caregiver: the emotional impact of the coronavirus epidemic on nurses and other health professionals". *Enfermería Clínica,* 1-5. https://doi.org/10.1016/j.enfcli.2020.05.006

- Cai H., Baoren T., Ma J., Chen L., Jiang Y., Zuhang Q. (2020). "Psychological. Impact and coping strategies of frontline health workers in Hunan between January and March 2020 during the 2019 outbreak of coronavirus disease (COVID-19) in Hubei, China". *Medical ScienceMonitor* , 26, 1-16. https://dx.doi.org/10.12659%2FMSM.924171

- Carlin, M. and Garcés de los Fayos Ruiz, E. J. (2010), "El síndrome de burnout: Evolución histórica desde el contexto laboral al ámbito deportivo", *Anales de Psychology,* 26(1), 169-180 ,available at : https:ZZwww.redalyc.orgZpdfZ167/16713758020.pdf

- Chartzman-Birenbaum, A. D. (2020), "Cuando los grises se pintan de blanco Acerca del fallo "Cáceres c. Provincia ART SA y Gobierno de la Ciudad de Buenos Aires s/amparo", *LA LEY.* Online-Zitat: ARZDOCZ1036Z2020.

- Chua S.E., Cheung V., Cheung C., et al. (2004), "Psychological Effects of the SARS Outbreak in Honq Konq on Hiqh-Risk Health Care Workers" [Psychological Impact of the SARS Outbreak in Hong Kong on Hiqh-Risk Health Care Workers]. *Can JPsychiatry* , 49 (6), 391-393. https:ZZdoi.orqZ10.1177%2F070674370404900609

- Firth-Cozens J. (2020), "What I learned from studying doctors' mental health over 20 years-an essay by Jenny Firth-Cozens", *British Medical Journal,* 369. https:ZZdoi.orqZ10.1136Zbmj.m1374

- Firth-Cozens J. and Greenhalgh J. (1997), "Doctors' perceptions of the links between stress and lowered clinical care", *Social Science & Medicine,* 44(7), 1017-1022. https:ZZdoi.orqZ10.1016ZS0277-9536(96)00227-4.

- Firth-Cozens J. and Cornwell J. (2009) 'Enabling compassionate care in acute care. Hospital settings" [Enabling compassionate care in acute hospital settings]. *King's Fund,* 1-16, available at: https:ZZwww.kinqsfund.orq.ukZsitesZdefaultZfilesZfieldZfieldpublicationfileZpoc-enabling-compassionate-care-hospital-settings-apr09.pdf.

- García-Moran, M., and Gil-Lacruz, M. (2016). "Stress in the Health care professionals." *Persona,* (19), 11-30, available at: https:ZZwww.redalyc.orqZpdfZ1471Z147149810001.pdf

- Gómez-Esteban, R. (2004), "El estrés laboral del médico: Burnout y trabajo en equipo". *Revista de la Asociación Española de Neuropsiquiatría,* (90), 41-56, available at: https:ZZwww.redalyc.orqZarticulo.oa?id=2650Z265019660004

- Grisolía, J.A. and Ahuad, E.J. (2019), *Riesgos del trabajo, guía práctica profesional,* Editorial Estudio.

- Lai J., Ma S., Wang Y., Cai Z., Hu J., Wei N. (2020), Factors Associated With Mental Health Outcomes Among Health Care Workers Exposed to Coronavirus Disease 2019. *JAMA Network Open* 3(3), 1-12. 10.1001/jamanetworkopen.2020.3976.

- Lee S.M., Kang W.S., Cho A., et al. (2018), "Psychological impact of the, 2015 MERS outbreak on hospital workers and quarantined hemodialysis patients", *Compr Psychiatry* 87, p. 123127. https://dx. doi.org/10.1016%2Fj.comppsych.2018.10.003

- Lozano-Vargas A. (2020), "Impact of the coronavirus epidemic (COVID-19). On the mental health of health workers and the general population in China". *RevistadeNeuro-Psiquiatria ,* 83(1), 51-56. https://doi.org/10.20453/rnp.v83i1.3687

- Martin, A. and Souto L. A. (2008), *Las nuevas enfermedades laborales: daño psíquico.* Induvio Editora.

    -Martínez-Pérez, A. (2010), "El síndrome de burnout. Conceptual development and The current state of the question", *Vivat Academia,* (112), 42-80. http://dx.doi.org/10.15178/va.2010.112.42-80

- Maunder R.G., Lancee W.J., Balderson K.E., et al. (2006), "Long-term Psychological and Occupational Effects of Providing Hospital Healthcare during SARS Outbreak", *Emerging Infectious Diseases,* 12 (12) 1924-1932. https://dx.doi.org/10.3201%2Feid1212.060584

- Molinaro, M. (2019), *Proceedings before judicial medical commissions. Law 27.348 and Res. 298/2017. teoría. Práctica y crítica,* Editorial García Alonso.

- Monterrosa-Castro A., Dávila-Ruiz R., Mejía-Mantilla A., Contreras-Saldarriaga J., Mercado-Lara M., and Flores-Monterrosa C. (2020) "Occupational stress, anxiety and fear of COVID-19 in Colombian general practitioners," *MedUNAB.* 23(2), 195213. https://doi.org/10.29375/01237047.3890. https://doi.org/10.29375/01237047.3890

- Montgomery A., Panagopoulou E., Esmail A., Richards T. and Maslach C. (2019), "Burnout in healthcare: the case for organisational change", *British Medical Journal,* 366. https://doi. org/10.1136/bmj.l4774

- National Institute of Mental Health (2020), "Post-traumatic stress disorder." *National Institutes of Health ,* (20), 1-8, available at: https://www.nimh.nih.gov/health/publications/espanol/trastorno-por-estres-	post-traumatic/20-mh-8124s-ptsd-sp 160750.pdf.

- International Labour Office (1984), "Psychosocial factors at work: nature, incidence and prevention," Occupational *Safety, Hygiene and Medicine,* (56), 1-85, available at: http://www.factorespsicosociales.com/wp-. Content/Uploads/2019/02/FPS-ILO-WHO.pdf

- O'Leary A., Jalloh M.F., Neria Y. (2018), 'Fear and culture: contextualising mental health impact of the 2014-2016 Ebola epidemic in West Africa'. *British Medical Journal Glob Health .* 3(3), 1-5. https://doi.org/10.1136/bmjgh-2018-000924. https://doi.org/10.1136/bmjgh-2018-000924

- Ovalles Pérez M.A. and Uribe Nobrega J.C. (2014), "Work-related stress, anxiety, and.

depresión en residentes de Medicina Interna y Cirugía General de un hospital público de Aragua", *Revista mexicana de salud del trabajo (REMESAT) ,* 6(16), 69-76, available at :https://fenastac.org.mx/wp-content/uploads/2015/02/REMESAT-EDICI%C3%93N-16.pdf

- International Labour Organization (2009), "Health and Life at Work: A Basic Human Right," *SafeDay*, 1, 1-18, available at: https://www.ilo.org/wcmsp5/groups/public/-edprotect/-protrav/---safework/documents/publication/wcms 151828.pdf

- International Labour Organization (2016), "Stress at work: a challenge for the future". Collective," *Safe Day*, 1, 1-68, available at: https://www.ilo.org/wcmsp5/groups/public/-edprotect/-protrav/---safework/documents/publication/wcms 466549.pdf

- International Labour Organization (2020), "ILO Standards and COVID-19. Frequently Asked Questions. Key provisions of international labour standards relevant in the context of the COVID-19 outbreak", 145, available at: https://www.ilo.org/wcmsp5/groups/public/---ednorm/---norms/documents/publication/wcms 739939.pdf.

- International Labour Organization and World Health Organization (2020), *Worker safety and health in health crises. Handbook on the protection of health workers and emergency teams,* ILO PRODOC, available at: https://www.ilo.org/wcmsp5/groups/public/-ed protect/---protrav/---safework/documents/publication/wcms 747129.pdf.

- World Health Organization (2004), "Work Organization and Stress: Systematic problem-solving strategies for employers, management and union representatives," *Protecting Workers' Health*, 3. 1-37, available at. https://www.who.int/occupational health/publications/pwh3en.pdf?ua=1

- Pan American Health Organization (2012), *Comparative study of working conditions and health of health workers in: Argentina, Brazil, Costa Rica and Peru,* Washington DC: PAHO/WHO, available at: https://www.paho.org/hq/dmdocuments/2012/HSS-Cond-Trab-RHS2012.pdf

- Pan American Health Organization (2013), "La salud de los trabajadores de la salud. Trabajo, empleo, organización y vida institucional en hospitales públicos del aglomerado Gran Buenos Aires, Argentina, 2010-2012," *Representación OPS/OMS Argentina,* 69, 1-244, available at: https://fesprosa.org.ar/portal/wp-content/uploads/2014/08/Salud-de-los-trabajadores-de-la-salud1 .pdf.

- Pan American Health Organization (2020), "Psychosocial and mental health considerations during the outbreak of COVID-19," *OPM/WHO,* 1-7, available at: https://www.paho.org/sites/default/files/2020-03/smaps-coronavirus-es-final-17- mar-20.pdf.

- Palacios-Nava, M.E., Morán-Álvarez I.C. and Paz-Román M. (2014), "Validación del inventario de Wolfgang en médicos mexicanos. Measurement of work stress in hospitals", *Revista mexicana de salud del trabajo (REMESAT)*, 6(16), 62-68, available at: https://fenastac.org.mx/wp-content/uploads/2015/02/REMESAT-EDICI%C3%93N-16.pdf.

- Quezada-Abascal, N. (2020), "The COVID-19, the protocols for health professionals and the right to refuse to work (Article 75 of the LCT)", *elDial.com.* Online citation: DC2A0A.

- Robbins, S.P. and Judge, T.A. (2009), *Comportamiento organizacional. Thirteenth edition,* Pearson Educación, Mexico.

- Romualdi E.E. (2020), *Ley de riesgos del trabajo. Prestaciones dinerarias. Trámites ante las Comisiones médicas,* Ed.

- Superintendencia de Riesgos del Trabajo (2017), *Medical and Expert Issues before the Courts in Occupational Accident and Occupational Disease Claims,* Academy for Exchange and Judicial Studies.

- Universidad Católica Boliviana San Pablo (2007), "El estrés laboral como síntoma de una empresa", *Perspectivas,* (20), 55-66, available at: https://www.redalyc.org/articulo.oa?id=4259/425942331005.

- Uribe-Prado, J., López-Flores P., Pérez-Galicia C. and García-Saisó, A. (2014), "Síndrome de Desgaste Ocupacional (Burnout) y su Relación con Salud y Riesgo Psicosocial en Funcionarios Públicos que Imparten Justicia en México, D.F.," *Acta de investigación psicológica,* 4(2), 1554-1571. https://doi.org/10.1016/S2007-4719(14)70393-X

- Xiang Y., Yang Y., Li W., Zhang L., Zhang Q., Cheung T., Chee H Ng. et al. (2020), "Timely mental health care for the 2019 novel coronavirus outbreak is urgently needed," 7(3), 228-229. https://doi.org/10.1016/S2215-0366(20)30046-8.

CONTENTS

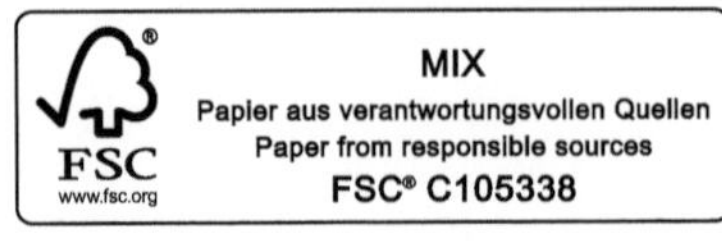

Printed by Books on Demand GmbH, Norderstedt / Germany